COMPLETE GUIDE TO UNDERSTANDING BREAST AUGMENTATION

Everything You Need To Know About Implants, Surgery Procedures, Costs, Risks, Recovery, And Achieving The Perfect Look

KLEIN HOYLE

Disclaimer

The content in this book is based on the author's expertise and comprehension of the topic. The author has no affiliation or link with any corporation, business, or person. This book is meant to give general information and educational material only, and it should not be interpreted as professional medical advice. Always seek the advice of a skilled healthcare expert if you have any queries about medical issues or treatments. The author and publisher expressly disclaim any responsibility resulting directly or indirectly from the use or use of the information included in this book.

Table of Contents

ABOUT THIS BOOK

"Complete Guide to Understanding Breast Augmentation" is a thorough resource that walks people through the complex process of breast augmentation. This book is more than just a handbook; it is a powerful tool meant to bring clarity, confidence, and thorough information to people contemplating or receiving breast augmentation surgery.

Chapter 1 looks into the fundamentals of breast augmentation, explaining the procedure's goals, advantages, and restrictions. It also presents alternate possibilities, allowing readers to make educated selections based on their preferences and circumstances. By setting the groundwork, readers may approach their trip with confidence and understanding.

Preparing for breast augmentation is a critical phase, which is thoroughly discussed in Chapter 2. From early meetings with surgeons to pre-operative testing and lifestyle changes, this chapter gives a road map for people to prepare physically, psychologically, and emotionally for the treatment. Such rigorous planning reduces risks and improves results.

Chapter 3 delves into the vast world of breast implants, informing readers of the many kinds, forms, textures, and sizes accessible. Understanding these variances enables people to make tailored decisions that are consistent with their aesthetic aspirations and anatomical concerns.

Choosing the correct surgeon is critical for a good result, as stressed in Chapter 4. Readers may choose a skilled surgeon who knows their vision and emphasizes their safety and happiness after doing thorough research, evaluating qualifications, and consulting with them.

Chapter 5 delves into the surgical route, including anesthetic choices, incision methods, implant placement, and predicted results. By demystifying the surgical process, readers acquire clarity and peace of mind, allowing them to go into the treatment with confidence.

Following surgery, Chapter 6 walks patients through the recovery process, including immediate care, pain management, follow-up visits, and resumption of normal activities. This chapter includes practical recommendations for a smooth and painless recovery while reducing stress and difficulties.

Chapter 7 frankly discusses the dangers and problems of breast augmentation, encouraging readers to spot warning signals and seek prompt treatment when needed. This chapter supports safety and well-being throughout the surgical process by raising awareness and preparing patients.

Chapter 8 covers post-operative care, including dressing instructions, medication management, physical limits, and supporting clothing. This chapter provides people with the information and skills they need to facilitate their recovery process and improve surgery results.

Long-term maintenance, as discussed in Chapter 9, stresses the necessity of monitoring breast health, knowing implant longevity, and being aware of possible issues. Individuals who prioritize long-term care and awareness may experience long-term contentment and peace of mind.

Finally, Chapter 10 discusses the psychological implications of breast augmentation, focusing on the road to self-acceptance, body image adjustment, and general confidence. By creating a supportive atmosphere and giving tools, this chapter ensures that people accept their new identities with grace and empowerment.

CHAPTER 1

Understanding Breast Augmentation

What Is Breast Augmentation?

Breast augmentation, commonly known as augmentation mammoplasty, is a surgical operation designed to improve the size, shape, and symmetry of a woman's breasts. This is accomplished by the use of breast implants or fat transfer procedures. The purpose of breast augmentation is to enhance the look of the breasts, giving patients more confidence and happiness with their body image.

The operation starts with a consultation with a trained plastic surgeon, during which the patient discusses their objectives, concerns, and expectations for breast augmentation. The surgeon assesses the patient's breast architecture, skin condition, and general health to decide the best method for getting the desired outcomes.

Breast implants are classified into three types: saline-filled, silicone gel-filled, and structured. The choice of implant is determined by several criteria, including the patient's body type, desired result, and the surgeon's advice. The implant may be placed submuscular (under the chest muscle) or subglandular (above the chest muscle), depending on the patient's anatomy and desire.

During surgery, incisions are made around the areola, in the inframammary fold (below the breast), or the armpit. The implants are then gently placed into the breast pockets made by the surgeon. After the implants have been placed and symmetrically adjusted, the incisions are sutured closed, and the breasts are bandaged in bandages or a surgical bra.

Reasons To Consider Breast Augmentation

Women choose breast augmentation for a variety of reasons, including aesthetics and reconstruction. Some frequent explanations are:

1. **Increasing breast size:** Many women want bigger breasts to obtain a more proportional and feminine appearance. Breast augmentation may enhance breast volume and improve body proportions.

2. **Improving breast shape:** Some women's breasts may be naturally asymmetrical or deformed, or they may have lost volume and firmness as a result of pregnancy, nursing, or weight loss. Breast augmentation may help you achieve a more youthful and beautiful breast shape.

3. **Boosting self-confidence:** Dissatisfaction with the size or form of one's breasts may affect a woman's self-esteem and body image.

Breast augmentation may offer a psychological boost by increasing the look of the breasts and general self-esteem.

4. Breast augmentation may also be used for breast reconstruction after mastectomy (the surgical removal of one or both breasts), trauma, or congenital defects. It aids in the restoration of breast form and volume, letting women reclaim their feeling of normality and femininity after breast cancer treatment or other medical procedures.

5. **Correcting developmental abnormalities:** Some women's breasts may be underdeveloped or congenital, affecting their physical appearance and self-esteem. Breast augmentation may assist with these difficulties, resulting in a more proportional and aesthetically acceptable breast form.

Advantages And Disadvantages Of Breast Augmentation

Breast augmentation has various advantages, including:

1. Breast augmentation may improve the overall balance and symmetry of the body, resulting in a more proportional and pleasing profile.

2. **Increased self-confidence:** After breast augmentation, many women report a gain in self-esteem and body image, feeling more comfortable and confident in their looks.

3. Breast augmentation is a highly customized surgery in which patients may choose the size, shape, and kind of implants that best fit their preferences and aesthetic objectives.

4. **Long-term results:** With appropriate care and maintenance, breast implants may improve the look of the breasts for many years.

However, it is important to recognize the limits and possible hazards of breast augmentation, which include:

1. Surgical hazards: Breast augmentation, like any other surgical operation, has risks such as infection, hemorrhage, anesthetic difficulties, and severe implant responses.

2. Implant-related problems: Although uncommon, issues include implant rupture, capsular contracture (hardening of the scar tissue surrounding the implant), implant displacement, and changes in breast feeling that may occur after breast augmentation.

3. Maintenance and follow-up: Breast implants may need future surgery for replacement or removal, and frequent follow-up sessions with a plastic surgeon are required to ensure the implants' health and integrity.

4. Potential for dissatisfaction: While many women are pleased with the outcomes of breast augmentation, others may be disappointed or dissatisfied owing to

unrealistic expectations, unexpected problems, or cosmetic issues.

Alternatives To Breast Augmentation

While breast augmentation is a popular and successful way to increase breast size and shape, there are other choices available for people who are not good candidates for surgery or prefer non-invasive therapies. Alternative alternatives to consider are:

1. A breast lift (mastopexy) is a surgical technique that lifts and reshapes drooping breasts without dramatically altering their size. It may be done alone or in combination with breast augmentation to produce the best results.

2. **Fat transfer breast augmentation:** This procedure involves removing fat from other parts of the body via liposuction and injecting it into the breasts to boost volume and contour. Fat transfer breast augmentation

provides a more natural-looking and comfortable alternative to standard breast implants.

3. Breast augmentation exercises: Exercises and methods such as chest presses, push-ups, and pectoral flies may assist in strengthening the chest muscles while also improving the look of the breasts. While these workouts may not considerably increase breast size, they may improve muscular tone and raise the breasts for a perkier look.

4. Breast enhancement creams and supplements: A variety of over-the-counter creams, lotions, and supplements are promoted as breast enhancers, with the promise of increasing breast size and firmness. However, the efficacy of these products is often questioned, and they may not provide substantial or long-term improvements.

5. Wearing padded bras or inserts may temporarily improve the look of the breasts by increasing volume and cleavage.

While these techniques give a non-invasive and reversible approach to get a larger bust, the results are not permanent.

Before considering any alternative to breast augmentation, you should speak with a knowledgeable healthcare expert about your objectives, concerns, and the acceptability of each treatment option. They can help you make an educated selection based on your specific requirements and preferences.

CHAPTER 2

Preparing For Breast Augmentation

Initial Consultation With A Surgeon

Before having breast augmentation surgery, it is important to arrange early consultations with a skilled specialist. These meetings provide a chance for you to discuss your objectives, concerns, and expectations for the process. During these appointments, the surgeon will assess your general health, medical history, and breast anatomy to decide if you are a good candidate for the procedure.

The first consultation also allows you to ask about any concerns you may have concerning the process, such as the many kinds of implants available, the surgical procedures employed, and the possible risks and issues involved. It's important to be upfront and honest with your surgeon about your goals and any medical issues you may have since this will allow them to create a unique treatment plan suited to your requirements.

In addition, the surgeon may measure your breasts and utilize imaging technologies to model the probable outcomes of the procedure. This gives you a better knowledge of what to anticipate after surgery and ensures that you and your physician agree on the intended result.

Finally, initial consultations with a surgeon are an important phase in the breast augmentation process since they allow you to collect information, address any concerns, and build rapport with your surgeon before proceeding with the treatment.

Pre-Operative Tests And Assessments

Before having breast augmentation surgery, you will need to go through several pre-operative tests and examinations to verify that you are in excellent health and that the procedure can be completed safely.

Depending on your age and medical history, these tests may include blood testing, a mammogram, an electrocardiogram (ECG), or other heart tests.

These tests are designed to detect any underlying health concerns that may raise the risks connected with surgery, such as blood disorders, heart ailments, or breast abnormalities. By recognizing these difficulties in advance, your surgeon may take the necessary steps to reduce the chance of complications during and after the treatment.

In addition to physical examinations, you may have a psychological evaluation to determine your mental and emotional fitness for surgery. This examination ensures that you have reasonable expectations for the procedure's outcome and that you are psychologically prepared to deal with the physical and emotional changes that may emerge from breast augmentation.

Overall, pre-operative examinations and evaluations are an important part of the breast augmentation process since they assure your safety and well-being before, during, and after the procedure.

Lifestyle Changes Before Surgery

To enhance your health and reduce the risk of problems before breast augmentation surgery, you should undertake specific lifestyle modifications. These changes may include stopping smoking, eating a balanced diet, and avoiding certain drugs and supplements that might raise the risk of bleeding or interfere with anesthetic.

Smoking is especially harmful to the healing process, increasing the risk of problems including infection and poor wound healing. As a result, it is highly advised that you stop smoking at least several weeks before surgery to give your body time to heal and recuperate.

Furthermore, eating a balanced diet rich in fruits, vegetables, lean meats, and whole grains will aid your immune system and encourage recovery.

It's also critical to keep hydrated by consuming lots of water in the days coming up to surgery.

Certain drugs and supplements, including aspirin, ibuprofen, and vitamin E, might thick the blood and raise the risk of bleeding after surgery. As a result, it's critical to follow your surgeon's directions for which drugs and supplements to avoid in the weeks preceding your treatment.

Making these lifestyle adjustments before surgery will help ensure a more comfortable recovery and better overall results following breast augmentation.

Mental Preparation For Surgery

Breast augmentation surgery may be an emotionally charged event, so take the time to psychologically prepare for the treatment and its possible effects. This might include addressing any worries or anxiety you have regarding surgery, as well as regulating your expectations about the outcome.

One method to psychologically prepare for surgery is to learn more about the operation and what to anticipate during the recovery period. This may help you overcome your worries and concerns while also giving you a feeling of control over the situation. Furthermore, speaking with friends or family members who have had comparable surgeries may give great support and insight.

It's also critical to care for your mental well-being in the days preceding surgery. This might include using relaxation methods like deep breathing exercises or meditation to help quiet your nerves and lessen tension.

Finally, it is critical to have reasonable expectations regarding the result of the procedure. While breast augmentation might improve the size and form of your breasts, it's vital to remember that no operation comes without dangers or limits. Having reasonable expectations can help you avoid disappointment and enjoy the outcomes of your operation.

CHAPTER 3

Types Of Breast Implants

Saline Vs Silicone Implants

There are two major kinds of breast implants available for augmentation surgery: saline and silicone. Each variety has unique traits and issues that patients should be aware of before making a selection.

Saline implants are filled with a sterile saltwater solution. They are usually placed empty and then filled with the proper size once in place. One benefit of saline implants is that if they burst, the saline solution is safely absorbed by the body. However, some patients report that saline implants feel less realistic than silicone implants and are more prone to apparent rippling or wrinkling.

Silicone implants, on the other hand, are filled with a cohesive silicone gel that has a texture similar to real breast tissue. Many patients report that silicone implants have a more natural appearance and feel than saline implants. Silicone implants are also less prone to ripple or wrinkle, especially in individuals who have thin skin or little natural breast tissue. However, if a silicone implant ruptures, the gel may remain inside the implant capsule or seep into the surrounding tissue, making detection more difficult than with a saline implant.

Finally, the decision between saline and silicone implants is based on the patient's specific preferences, anatomy, and intended goals. Patients should explore the advantages and disadvantages of each choice with their surgeon to decide which kind of implant is most suited to their requirements.

Round Vs Teardrop-Shaped Implants

When it comes to breast augmentation, patients may select between round or teardrop-shaped implants, each with its own set of qualities and benefits.

Round implants are the most often utilized breast implants in augmentation surgery. As the name implies, these implants have a symmetrical, rounded form that adds fullness and projection to the breasts. Round implants are adaptable and may boost both the upper and lower poles of the breasts, giving them a more enhanced look. They are also less costly than teardrop-shaped implants, and they come in a variety of sizes and shapes to suit varied patient needs.

Teardrop-shaped implants, sometimes called anatomical or contoured implants, provide a more natural appearance and closely mirror the form of a natural breast. These implants have a tapering top and a broader bottom, replicating the breast's natural slope. Teardrop-shaped implants are often favored by individuals who want a more modest enlargement or have little natural breast tissue. However, they must be carefully placed to retain their appropriate alignment and avoid rotation, which might result in an asymmetrical look.

Finally, the decision between round and teardrop-shaped implants is based on the patient's desired result, anatomy, and personal preferences. Patients should discuss their objectives with their physician to identify which implant form is most suited to attain the desired outcomes.

Textured Vs Smooth Implants

Breast implants have two surface textures: textured and smooth. Each kind of surface texture has distinct qualities and advantages that should be carefully evaluated when selecting the appropriate implant for breast augmentation surgery.

Textured implants feature a rough surface that is intended to attach to the surrounding tissue, lowering the likelihood of implant rotation or displacement. This is especially useful for teardrop-shaped implants, which need precision positioning to retain their natural orientation. Textured implants also have a decreased chance of capsular contracture, a condition in which scar tissue accumulates around the implant, making the breast feel stiff or deformed. However, some patients may notice that textured implants have a somewhat stiffer sensation than smooth implants.

Smooth implants have a smooth surface, which permits them to move more easily within the breast pocket. This may provide a softer, more natural sensation than textured implants. Smooth implants are also less prone to cause rippling or wrinkles, especially in individuals with thin skin or little natural breast tissue. However, they may have a little increased risk of capsular contracture than textured implants.

Finally, the decision between textured and smooth implants is based on the patient's unique anatomy, preferences, and intended goals. Patients must examine the advantages and disadvantages of each choice with their surgeon to choose which kind of implant surface texture is most suited to their requirements.

Implant Sizes And Profiles

Selecting the appropriate implant size and profile is one of the most important considerations in breast augmentation surgery. Implant size refers to the implant's volume, which is measured in cubic centimeters (cc) or milliliters (ml), while implant profile refers to the implant's protrusion from the chest wall.

The implant size should be carefully chosen based on the patient's body proportions, chest breadth, breast base diameter, and desired result. When determining the proper implant size, patients should take into account their lifestyle, activity level, and wardrobe choices. It is critical to talk freely with the surgeon about the desired cup size and aesthetic objectives to guarantee that the implant size selected delivers the desired result.

The implant profile influences how far the breasts protrude from the chest wall. Implants come in a variety of profiles, including low, moderate, high, and very high. The implant's profile should be determined by the patient's anatomy, existing breast tissue, and desired amount of projection. For example, patients with a small chest width may benefit from a higher profile implant to produce greater projection, while patients with a wider chest may choose a lower profile implant for a more natural appearance.

During the consultation, the surgeon will thoroughly assess the patient's anatomy and describe the different implant sizes and profiles available. They may also employ 3D imaging technology to simulate various implant sizes and forms, letting the patient see possible results before making a final selection.

Determining the appropriate implant size and profile requires careful evaluation of the patient's anatomy, objectives, and preferences.

CHAPTER 4

Selecting The Right Surgeon

Researching And Choosing A Qualified Surgeon

Choosing the appropriate physician for your breast augmentation is critical to getting the results you want and keeping the process safe. Begin by looking for doctors in your region that specialize in breast augmentation. To identify possible candidates, go through internet resources such as medical directories and review websites. Additionally, get suggestions from friends or family members who have had comparable treatments.

Once you've compiled a list of probable surgeons, extensively investigate each of them. Look for information about their education, training, certifications, and previous experience with breast augmentation surgeries. Board certification in plastic surgery is strong evidence of a surgeon's ability and dedication to providing high-quality patient care.

It's also vital to examine the surgeon's standing in the medical community. Look for any disciplinary proceedings or malpractice claims filed against the surgeon, as well as good recommendations from peers or professional organizations.

Evaluating Surgeon Credentials And Experience

When reviewing a surgeon's qualifications and expertise, pay special attention to their track record of breast augmentation surgeries. Inquire about how many augmentations they have done and seek to view before-and-after images of past patients. This can help you have a better understanding of the surgeon's aesthetic approach and competence level.

In addition to technical competence, think about the surgeon's attitude to patient care. Are they listening and responding to your inquiries and concerns? Do they take the time to properly explain the operation and discuss any possible risks or complications? A skilled surgeon should stress open communication and keep you comfortable and informed during the procedure.

Consultation With Surgeon

Before making a final choice, meet with the surgeon to discuss your objectives and expectations for breast augmentation. This is a time for you to ask any concerns you may have regarding the surgery and determine if you feel comfortable and confident with the surgeon.

During the appointment, the surgeon will examine your anatomy and discuss breast implant alternatives, incision location, and surgical procedures. They should also set realistic expectations for the procedure's outcomes, including any possible risks or problems.

Inquire about the surgeon's approach to postoperative care and follow-up sessions. A professional surgeon will have a detailed strategy in place to ensure your recuperation goes smoothly and successfully.

Patient Reviews And Testimonials

In addition to investigating the surgeon's qualifications and expertise, reading patient reviews and testimonials may give useful information about the kind of care you can anticipate. Look for evaluations from people who have had breast augmentation with the surgeon you are considering, and pay special attention to their overall happiness with the outcomes and their experience during the procedure.

While favorable evaluations might be encouraging, it's equally crucial to weigh any negative comments or concerns expressed by former patients.

Look for trends or repeated themes in the evaluations that might be warning flags, such as poor communication, hasty consultations, or unsatisfying results.

Finally, selecting the best surgeon for your breast augmentation is a personal choice that should be founded on extensive study, thoughtful analysis of your alternatives, and confidence in your selected physician. By taking the time to consider surgeon qualifications, expertise, and patient feedback, you may be confident in your selection and look forward to accomplishing your goals.

CHAPTER 5

The Breast Augmentation Procedure

Anesthesia Options

Anesthesia is an essential component of all surgical procedures, including breast augmentation. General anesthesias, local anesthesia with sedation, and, in rare cases, regional anesthesia are commonly accessible choices. The decision is determined by several criteria, including the patient's health, the surgeon's preference, and the difficulty of the procedure.

General anesthesia is often used for breast augmentation procedures because it enables the patient to remain asleep and painless during the surgery. This entails administering drugs that cause a transient state of unconsciousness. To guarantee the patient's safety during surgery, an anesthesiologist closely checks their vital signs.

Another alternative is local anesthesia with sedation, which involves the surgeon numbing the breast region with a local anesthetic while the patient remains aware but comfortable owing to the sedative. This option may be appropriate for some individuals or less invasive treatments.

Regional anesthetic, such as epidural or nerve blocks, may be used in certain situations to numb particular parts of the body and relieve pain during and after surgery. However, it is less typically utilized for breast augmentation than other forms of surgery.

Before surgery, the anesthesiologist will go over the alternatives with the patient, taking into consideration their medical history, allergies, and preferences. The objective is to choose the most suitable anesthetic option for a pleasant and safe surgical experience.

Incision Placement Techniques

The incision placement strategy used in breast augmentation surgery has a substantial impact on scarring, implant placement, and overall surgical results. Inframammary, periareolar, transaxillary, and transumbilical incisions are among the most common.

The inframammary incision is performed following the natural crease behind the breast, where the scar is usually well disguised. This method enables direct access to the breast tissue, allowing for accurate implant implantation.

Periareolar incisions are done along the edge of the areola, where the shift in pigmentation helps to conceal the scar. This approach is appropriate for patients who want to leave as little scarring as possible, and it may also help with some kinds of implant placement.

Transaxillary incisions are done in the underarm region to enable implant implantation without leaving obvious scars on the breast. However, this procedure may be more difficult for the surgeon and not appropriate for all implant types.

Transumbilical incisions, also known as TUBA (transumbilical breast augmentation), require creating a surgical incision around the belly button to insert and position the implants into the breast pocket. While this treatment produces no visible scars on the breast, it is only suited for saline implants and needs specialist surgical skills.

During the consultation, the surgeon will discuss the benefits and drawbacks of each incision placement approach with the patient, taking into consideration aspects such as implant type, desired goals, and individual preferences.

Implant Placement Options: Submuscular Vs. Subglandular

One of the most important considerations in breast augmentation surgery is where to put the implants in the chest muscles and the breast tissue. There are two main options: submuscular (under the chest muscle) and sub-glandular (below the breast tissue but above the muscle).

Submuscular implant placement entails placing the implants under the pectoral muscles. This placement gives extra covering and support for the implants, resulting in a more natural appearance and a lower likelihood of noticeable rippling. It may also make mammograms simpler to read.

Subglandular implant placement, on the other hand, requires placing the implants beneath the breast tissue but above the chest muscles. This location may result in a somewhat faster recovery since the chest muscles are not affected during surgery. However, subglandular implants may be more apparent, particularly in individuals with thin breast tissue, and there is a somewhat increased risk of capsular contracture.

During the consultation, the surgeon will assess the patient's anatomy, breast features, and cosmetic aspirations to determine the best implant placement choice. This selection will be influenced by factors such as breast size, shape, and natural breast tissue content.

Surgical Duration And Expected Results

The length of breast augmentation surgery depends on several variables, including the procedure's intricacy, the surgical method used, and if any other operations are done concurrently (such as a breast lift). Breast augmentation surgery normally lasts one to two hours.

Patients should anticipate swelling, bruising, and soreness in the days after surgery, but these symptoms will progressively reduce with time.

Most patients may resume work and mild activities within a week, but excessive activity and heavy lifting should be avoided for a few weeks to allow for adequate recovery.

The ultimate outcomes of breast augmentation surgery may not be seen right away owing to edema and early post-operative alterations. However, once the swelling goes down and the breasts adjust to their new form, patients will see a considerable improvement in breast size, shape, and overall look.

Patients must carefully follow their surgeon's post-operative recommendations to achieve maximum healing and long-term outcomes. Regular follow-up consultations will let the surgeon evaluate progress, resolve any concerns, and ensure that the patient is satisfied with the result.

CHAPTER 6

Recovery Process

Immediate Post-Operative Care

Immediate post-operative care is critical for a healthy recovery after breast augmentation surgery. After the treatment, you will be sent to a recovery room where medical personnel will check your vital signs and make sure you are comfortable. It is common to feel some discomfort and grogginess shortly after surgery as a result of the anesthetic, but your medical team will prescribe appropriate pain management medicine to reduce any discomfort.

Your breasts will most likely be covered in bandages or a surgical bra to give support and reduce swelling. To avoid infection, follow your surgeon's wound care recommendations, which include keeping the incision areas clean and dry. Antibiotics may also be prescribed to lower your infection risk.

During the early recuperation phase, it is critical to relax and avoid hard activity or heavy lifting. Your body needs time to heal, so take it easy and let yourself recuperate completely before resuming your usual schedule.

Pain Management Techniques

Effective pain management is an important part of the healing process after breast augmentation surgery. Your surgeon will prescribe pain medication to assist relieve any discomfort you may have in the days after surgery. It is critical to take these drugs as prescribed and not exceed the authorized dose.

In addition to medicine, there are additional methods you may use to alleviate pain and promote recovery. Ice packs may help minimize swelling and pain in your breasts, particularly in the first 48 hours following surgery. To avoid damaging your skin, cover the ice packs in a towel.

Maintaining good posture and avoiding exercises that strain your chest muscles may also assist in alleviating pain and discomfort. Sleeping with your upper body raised on pillows might help to minimize edema and drain excess fluid from the surgery site.

Follow-Up Appointments And Monitoring

Following breast augmentation surgery, you should schedule follow-up sessions with your surgeon to check your progress and verify that your breasts are healing appropriately. These consultations are an important part of the healing process because they enable your surgeon to evaluate the outcome of the operation and address any concerns or difficulties that may emerge.

During these follow-up meetings, your surgeon will check your breasts, remove any bandages or stitches, and talk about your healing progress. They may also conduct further tests or imaging examinations to assess the surgical success and rule out any problems, such as infection or implant displacement.

Attend all planned follow-up visits and speak honestly with your surgeon about any symptoms or concerns you may have. Your surgeon will be present for you throughout your recuperation and will work with you to resolve any concerns that occur.

Resuming Regular Activities And Exercise

As you recuperate, you will eventually be able to return to your usual daily activities and exercise program. However, you must listen to your body and avoid pushing yourself too hard too quickly. Your surgeon will advise you on when it is safe to resume certain activities depending on your specific healing status.

Initially, you should avoid any activities that require heavy lifting or severe activity, since they might strain your chest muscles and interfere with the healing process. Begin cautiously with simple exercises like walking and progressively raise the intensity as you feel comfortable.

When it comes to exercise, it's important to ease back into your routine and avoid exercises that place too much pressure on your chest muscles, such as weightlifting or high-impact aerobics. Low-impact workouts like walking, swimming, and yoga may help with healing since they enhance circulation and flexibility while placing little strain on your breasts.

Remember to always follow your surgeon's advice and listen to your body throughout the healing period. By taking care of yourself and giving yourself enough time to recuperate, you can secure the greatest possible result from your breast augmentation surgery.

CHAPTER 7

Risks And Complications

Common Risks Associated With Breast Augmentation

Breast augmentation, like other surgical procedures, has inherent dangers. Understanding the risks is critical for anybody contemplating surgery. Infection is a frequent danger. Although uncommon, infections may arise after surgery, resulting in problems that may need extra treatment. Another danger is capsular contracture, which occurs when scar tissue grows around the implant, making the breast feel stiff or deformed. This may be unpleasant and may need corrective surgery.

Hematoma and seroma are other possible hazards. Hematomas are blood collections that may form around the implant site, while seromas are fluid collections that look similar. Both may cause pain, and edema and may need drainage. Furthermore, breast augmentation may cause changes in nipple feeling or breast asymmetry. While some alterations may fade with time, others may need further intervention.

Patients should address these hazards with their surgeon to better understand their unique risk factors. Smoking, obesity, and certain medical problems all raise the risk of complications. Patients may make educated surgical choices if they understand the risks and take the necessary safeguards.

Potential Complications During And Following Surgery

Several issues might occur with breast augmentation surgery. One such consequence is anesthesia-related problems. Anesthesia responses are infrequent but may range from moderate nausea to more serious consequences. Careful supervision by a competent anesthesiologist may assist to reduce these dangers.

Another possible hazard is bleeding during or after the operation. Excessive bleeding may cause hematomas, which may need extra intervention for management. Proper surgical technique and post-operative surveillance may significantly decrease the incidence of bleeding problems.

Implant problems, including rupture or leaking, may occur during or after surgery. Modern implants are intended to be lasting, yet they are not invincible. Regular monitoring and follow-up meetings with your surgeon may help discover problems early and avoid consequences.

Signs Of Complications To Watch For

After breast augmentation surgery, it is critical to watch for symptoms of problems. One typical symptom is increased pain or discomfort that is not alleviated by pain medication. Swelling, redness, or warmth at the incision site may suggest infection and should be reported to your surgeon right once.

Similarly, if you detect any changes in the look or feel of your breasts, such as asymmetry or distortion, get medical assistance right once.

Other indicators of problems include fever, chills, or flu-like symptoms, which might suggest an underlying infection. Any changes in nipple feeling, such as numbness or tingling, should be reported to your surgeon. While some soreness and swelling are expected following surgery, any persistent or severe symptoms should be handled right once to avoid potential issues.

When To Contact Your Surgeon

Knowing when to call your surgeon is critical for a successful recovery and reducing the risk of complications. If you notice any of the symptoms listed above, such as increasing discomfort, swelling, redness, or changes in nipple feeling, you should call your surgeon immediately. Prompt treatment may help keep issues from worsening and may need further intervention.

Additionally, if you have any issues or questions concerning your healing process, do not hesitate to contact your surgeon. They are available to help you during your trip and may provide advice and reassurance as required. Remember that your health and safety are the most important considerations, so do not hesitate to seek medical assistance if you have any concerns regarding your recovery after breast augmentation surgery.

CHAPTER 8

Postoperative Care

Dressing And Wound Care Instructions

Proper dressing and wound care are essential after breast augmentation surgery to promote healing and reduce the risk of infection. Your surgeon will give you specific recommendations based on your unique condition, but here are some broad suggestions to follow.

First and foremost, your incision sites will most likely be covered with dressings or bandages. It is critical to maintain these dressings dry and sanitary. Your surgeon may advise you to change them regularly or to wait until your first follow-up session before removing them. If you observe any bleeding, unusual discharge, or symptoms of infection around the incisions, such as increased redness, edema, or warmth, you should call your surgeon immediately.

In addition, you may be told to wear a surgical bra or compression garment to support your breasts and reduce swelling. It's critical to follow your surgeon's instructions for wearing these garments and when you may switch to ordinary bras.

As your wounds heal, you may experience itching or pain. It is critical to avoid scratching or picking at the incisions since they may disturb the healing process and increase the risk of infection or scarring. To encourage healing and limit the chance of scarring, your surgeon may prescribe using mild cleansers or ointments for your wounds.

Throughout the healing process, it is critical to closely follow your surgeon's instructions and attend all planned follow-up visits. Your surgeon will monitor your progress, remove any sutures or drains as required, and handle any concerns or issues that may occur.

By following correct dressing and wound care guidelines, you may help guarantee a smooth recovery and the best possible outcomes from your breast augmentation procedure.

Medication Management After Surgery

Following breast augmentation surgery, your surgeon will most likely prescribe medicine to alleviate discomfort and limit the chance of infection. It is critical that you carefully follow your surgeon's instructions and take any prescription medicines exactly as indicated.

Pain management is an important part of your rehabilitation process. To assist reduce discomfort in the first few days following surgery, your surgeon may prescribe pain medicines. It is critical to take these drugs as prescribed and not wait until the pain gets severe before taking them. Staying ahead of the pain allows you to better manage discomfort and encourage a speedier recovery.

In addition to pain relievers, your surgeon may recommend antibiotics to lower the chance of infection. It is critical to take these drugs precisely as prescribed, even if you begin to feel better before completing the complete course. Failure to finish the authorized course of medicines increases the risk of illness or antibiotic resistance.

In addition to prescription drugs, your surgeon may offer over-the-counter pain relievers or anti-inflammatory medications to alleviate discomfort and swelling. It is important to check with your surgeon before taking any new drugs, since some may mix with your current medications or raise the risk of problems.

Throughout the healing process, you should discuss freely with your surgeon about any concerns or adverse effects from your medicines. Your surgeon might change your medication regimen as required to keep you comfortable and safe throughout the healing process.

Physical Restriction And Limitations

Following breast augmentation surgery, it is essential to follow physical restrictions and limits to encourage normal healing and reduce the risk of problems. Your surgeon will offer precise instructions depending on your unique situation, but here are some basic limitations to anticipate.

In the days and weeks after surgery, you should avoid intense activity and heavy lifting. This includes activities like weightlifting, hauling big bags, and rigorous exercise. These activities may put pressure on surgical wounds, increasing the risk of problems including bleeding or implant displacement.

Your surgeon may also suggest that you avoid sleeping positions or postures that exert strain on your breasts. Sleeping on your back with your upper body raised may assist relieve swelling and pain while also promoting appropriate recovery.

It's important to listen to your body and avoid activities or motions that cause pain or discomfort. If you're unclear if a specific activity is safe during your recuperation, it's advisable to be cautious and check with your surgeon.

As you recuperate, your surgeon may progressively remove or adjust physical limits according to your progress and healing. It is critical to follow your surgeon's instructions attentively and not hurry the healing process. Allowing your body enough time to recuperate can assist achieve the greatest possible outcomes from your breast augmentation surgery.

Support Garments And Bras

Following breast augmentation surgery, wearing suitable support garments and bras is critical for good healing and achieving the desired outcomes. Your surgeon will most likely make particular suggestions depending on your unique situation, but here are some broad guidelines to anticipate.

In the immediate aftermath of surgery, you will most likely be recommended to wear a surgical bra or compression garment to support your breasts and reduce swelling. These garments serve to anchor the implants, decrease movement, and offer mild compression that promotes healing.

As you recuperate, your surgeon may suggest switching to a soft, supportive sports bra or a wireless bra. It's critical to choose a bra that offers enough support while avoiding strain on surgical incisions or implants. Underwire bras should be avoided during the first few weeks after recovery because they might irritate the incisions and slow healing.

Your surgeon may also suggest that you wear a supportive bra at night to assist in maintaining appropriate breast position and prevent pain while sleeping. It is critical to follow your surgeon's instructions for when and how long to wear supporting garments and bras throughout your rehabilitation.

Attending all planned follow-up sessions with your surgeon is critical throughout the healing process. Your surgeon will track your progress, evaluate the healing of your incisions, and advise you on when you may switch to conventional bras and resume normal activities.

By adhering to your surgeon's recommendations for support garments and bras, you may assist in guaranteeing a smooth recovery and the best potential outcomes after breast augmentation surgery.

CHAPTER 9

Long-Term Maintenance

Monitoring Breast Health

Individuals who have had breast augmentation surgery need regular monitoring of their breast health. This involves doing self-examinations at home and arranging frequent appointments with a healthcare professional. Self-examinations consist of visually evaluating the breasts for changes in size, shape, or texture, as well as feeling for lumps or anomalies. These tests must be performed regularly, and any problems should be reported to a healthcare physician as soon as possible.

In addition to self-examinations, patients should schedule frequent follow-up sessions with their plastic surgeon. During these sessions, the surgeon will examine the implants, look for symptoms of problems, and answer any concerns or questions the patient may have. These consultations provide a chance to confirm that the implants are working well and that no problems necessitate addressing.

Breast health monitoring also entails maintaining up-to-date on any new advances or studies about breast implants and their possible influence on health. This involves being informed of any recalls or warnings made by regulatory bodies, as well as remaining current on the most recent guidelines for breast health and implant care.

Implant Lifespan And Possible Replacements

Breast implants are not intended to last a lifetime, and patients need to understand the lifespan of their implants and when they may need to be replaced. While the precise lifetime of breast implants varies based on the kind of implant used as well as individual characteristics such as age and lifestyle, the majority of implants are predicted to survive between 10 and 20 years.

As implants age, they may become more susceptible to problems like rupture, leakage, or capsular contracture. Furthermore, changes in breast tissue over time, such as weight fluctuations or pregnancy, might alter the look and feel of the implants. This is why people need to be aware of the indicators that their implants may need to be changed, such as changes in breast form or size, discomfort or pain, or obvious evidence of implant degradation.

Individuals may examine their alternatives for replacing breast implants with their plastic surgeon. This might include selecting a different kind or size of implant, as well as resolving any concerns or complications that have occurred following the first operation. Revision surgery to replace breast implants may help people retain the look and feel of their breasts over time, allowing them to feel confident and content with their results.

Breast Implant Illness (Bii) Awareness

Breast implant illness (BII) refers to a set of symptoms that some people ascribe to their breast implants. These symptoms might range from weariness to physical discomfort, cognitive difficulties, and more. While the actual etiology of BII is unknown, some experts think that particular materials or components of breast implants may elicit an immunological reaction in certain patients, resulting in these symptoms.

Individuals contemplating breast augmentation surgery should be informed of the hazards connected with breast implants, including the chance of BII. While the prevalence of BII is minimal, it is nevertheless important to take any concerns or symptoms seriously and get medical attention if needed. This might include talking with a healthcare practitioner to evaluate the source of symptoms and explore possible treatment choices.

Individuals who feel they have BII symptoms may benefit from revision surgery to remove or replace breast implants. However, it is important to contact with a trained healthcare expert before making this choice, as they can give individualized counsel and assistance based on particular circumstances.

Revision Surgery Considerations

Individuals who develop issues or alterations in their breast implants may need revision surgery. This might include implant rupture, capsular contracture, changes in breast form or size, or unhappiness with the original surgical outcomes. Revision surgery entails removing or replacing existing implants, as well as resolving any additional problems or complications that have occurred after the first operation.

Before having revision surgery, patients should discuss their concerns and objectives with their plastic surgeon. This may include assessing the status of current implants, discussing prospective adjustments to implant size or type, and addressing any other considerations that may influence the surgery's result. Individuals should have reasonable expectations regarding the consequences of revision surgery and accept that the intended outcome is not always feasible.

Insurance may fund revision surgery if it is considered medically necessary. However, this may differ based on individual insurance coverage and the grounds for the revision operation. Individuals should consult with their insurance provider to discover what is covered and address any financial concerns with their plastic surgeon.

Overall, revision surgery may help people preserve the look and feel of their breasts over time while also addressing any concerns or complications that may occur after breast augmentation surgery. Individuals may maintain their confidence and satisfaction with their breast augmentation outcomes by being knowledgeable about the possibility of requiring revision surgery and working closely with their plastic surgeon.

CHAPTER 10

Lifestyle Changes And Body Confidence

The Psychological Effects Of Breast Augmentation

Beginning the path of breast augmentation is about more than just the physical alteration; it is also about comprehending the psychological consequences. Many people choose breast augmentation because they want to improve their self-esteem and physical image. However, it is critical to understand that the psychological impacts differ from individual to person.

One typical psychological consequence is a boost in self-esteem. Many people report feeling more confident and good about their looks after having breast augmentation. This increase in self-esteem may have far-reaching consequences, affecting how individuals behave in social settings and even their general quality of life.

However, it is critical to approach breast augmentation with reasonable expectations. While it may improve physical appearance, it is not a panacea for underlying concerns such as self-esteem or body image. To have the greatest potential result, any underlying psychological problems must be addressed before surgery.

Another psychological factor to consider is the likelihood of emotional adjustment after surgery. It is typical to feel a variety of emotions throughout the rehabilitation process, such as enthusiasm, worry, and even periods of uncertainty. This transition phase is a normal part of the path to a new body image and should be handled with care and understanding.

Adjusting to Your New Body Image

Many people struggle to adapt to their new body image after having breast augmentation surgery. This process may be both exhilarating and frustrating as they figure out how their changing look fits into their sense of self.

One component of adapting to a new body image is learning to accept and enjoy the changes. This might be changing your outfit to fit your new shape or just taking the time to enjoy your improved contours. It is important to concentrate on the benefits and remind yourself of the reasons for your choice to get breast augmentation.

At the same time, it is common to have periods of doubt or hesitation throughout the transition phase. Allow yourself the time and space you need to gradually adjust to your new body image. Surrounding oneself with supportive friends and family may also help make the adjustment easier and give comfort during times of uneasiness.

Maintaining Total Body Confidence

While breast augmentation might increase self-confidence, it is important to realize that genuine body confidence extends beyond physical attractiveness. Maintaining general body confidence entails accepting all parts of oneself, both inside and out.

Practicing self-care and prioritizing your physical and emotional well-being is one method to boost body confidence. This might include getting regular exercise, practicing mindfulness and self-compassion, and surrounding oneself with good influences.

It's also important to create a positive connection with your body, treating it with compassion and respect. This includes avoiding using negative self-talk or comparing yourself to unreasonable expectations.

Instead, appreciate your body for what it can achieve and the adventure it has brought you on.

Support Groups And Resources For Breast Augmentation Patients

Navigating the breast augmentation process may be daunting at times, which is why having a solid support network is essential. Whether it's friends, family, or other patients, having people who understand and support your choice may make all the difference.

In addition to personal support networks, breast augmentation patients may use a variety of services. This might include internet forums, support groups, or instructional materials created by plastic surgeons. These sites may provide helpful insights, guidance, and encouragement at all stages of the process.

Furthermore, it is critical to have open contact with your cosmetic surgeon and healthcare staff. They may provide specialized advice and assistance based on your unique requirements and concerns. Remember that you are not alone on this journey, and there are several tools available to help you feel educated, empowered, and confident along the way.

Conclusion

Finally, comprehending breast augmentation entails more than just the desire for physical alteration; it also dives into the complexities of personal empowerment, body image, and the link between self-perception and cultural beauty standards. Throughout this thorough guide, we have looked at all areas of breast augmentation surgery, from early planning to surgical techniques and post-operative care.

One of the main lessons is the significance of doing extensive research and consulting with experienced medical practitioners. Breast augmentation is a serious choice that should be carefully considered, both physically and emotionally. Patients who visit with board-certified plastic surgeons may learn important information about the treatment, reasonable expectations, and possible risks and problems.

Furthermore, knowing the many kinds of breast implants, surgical procedures, and incision alternatives enables people to make educated decisions that reflect their cosmetic objectives and lifestyle preferences. Whether you choose saline or silicone implants, submuscular or subglandular implantation, or periareolar or inframammary incisions, be sure you understand the benefits and drawbacks of each choice.

Furthermore, understanding the significance of pre-operative preparation and post-operative care is critical for achieving optimum results and reducing the risk of problems. Patients take an active part in their rehabilitation, from maintaining a healthy lifestyle and stopping smoking to strictly adhering to post-operative instructions.

Aside from the physical benefits, breast augmentation may have a significant psychological impact on self-confidence and self-esteem. For many people, increasing their breast size or form may raise their confidence and improve their body image, resulting in a stronger feeling of self-assurance and contentment with how they look.

However, it is critical to understand that breast augmentation is not a cure-all for underlying self-esteem problems or body dysmorphia. While it may improve physical attractiveness, genuine confidence, and self-acceptance come from the inside and are not dependent on outward factors.

Finally, comprehending breast augmentation requires a comprehensive approach that takes into account physical, emotional, and psychological factors. Individuals may confidently and empoweredly begin their breast augmentation journey by equipping themselves with information, getting help from skilled specialists, and keeping reasonable expectations. Finally, whether you choose to get surgery or accept natural beauty, the most essential thing is to cultivate a good body image and self-love that goes beyond conventional expectations and celebrates originality.

THE END